COMPLETE GUIDE TO GLUCOSE

The Power of Eliminating Cravings and Balancing Blood Sugar Level

Nancy Cally

TABLE OF CONTENTS

INTRODUCTION

We explore the complex world of blood sugar control, cravings management, and the significant effects these variables have on your health and well-being in "The Ultimate Glucose Guide: The Power of Eliminating Cravings and Balancing Blood Sugar Levels." For the best energy, emotional stability, and general health, blood sugar levels must remain balanced. Finding and maintaining this balance may be difficult, however, given the processed meals, sedentary lifestyle, and high levels of stress associated with contemporary living.

This book serves as your road map for comprehending the mechanics of blood sugar regulation and equipping you with useful tactics to get rid of cravings and regulate your blood sugar levels. The tips and methods in this book will be very helpful whether you are trying to manage your diabetes, increase your energy, or just lead a healthy lifestyle.

Come along on this life-changing adventure with us as we examine the science behind blood sugar management, identify the underlying reasons for cravings, and provide you with practical strategies for managing your glucose levels. Together, let's set out on a journey to sustained well-being, happier moods, and abundant energy.

CHAPTER 1

THE VALUE OF BLOOD SUGAR LEVEL BALANCE

Maintaining glucose levels, or balanced blood sugar levels, is essential for general health and well-being. Blood sugar levels must be regulated for the following main reasons:

1. **Energy Regulation:** The main energy source for the cells in your body, particularly the brain, is glucose. A regulated blood sugar prevents the highs and crashes that come with blood sugar swings, giving you consistent energy levels all day long.

2. **Mood Stability:** Blood sugar abnormalities might impact your mental state and mood. Low blood sugar may induce anxiety, trouble focusing, and even melancholy. High blood sugar can cause irritation, mood changes, and

weariness. A more steady and upbeat mood is supported by maintaining regulated glucose levels.

3. **Weight Management:** Maintaining a healthy blood sugar balance is essential for controlling weight and avoiding obesity. Excess glucose may be transformed and stored as fat during blood sugar rises. Conversely, persistently low blood sugar levels might cause an increase in hunger and desire for items rich in calories or sugar.

4. **Diabetes Management:** It's critical to keep blood sugar levels in check for those with diabetes. Controlling blood sugar levels properly helps avoid consequences including renal disease, nerve damage, eyesight difficulties, and cardiovascular problems. It also lessens the need for insulin injections and prescription drugs.

5. **Heart Health:** Blood sugar swings might affect heart health. Elevated blood sugar levels raise the risk of heart disease, stroke, and other cardiovascular disorders by causing inflammation, insulin resistance, and arterial damage. Stable blood glucose levels promote heart health.

6. **Stable Energy Levels:** Throughout the day, stable energy levels are a result of balanced blood sugar levels. This stability improves your general quality of life and performance in day-to-day tasks by keeping you awake, focused, and productive.

7. **Prevention of Metabolic illnesses:** Insulin resistance and metabolic syndrome are two examples of metabolic illnesses that may be prevented by long-term blood sugar abnormalities. You may lessen your chance of developing these disorders and support

metabolic health by keeping your blood glucose levels in check.

To sum up, stable moods, energy, proper weight management, diabetes control, heart health, and general well-being all depend on having regulated blood sugar levels. You may experience prolonged vitality and longevity by implementing lifestyle practices that promote glucose balance, such as a nutritious diet, consistent exercise, stress reduction, and enough sleep.

The Effects of Cravings on Vitality and Health

Energy levels and physical health may both be significantly impacted by cravings, particularly for sugary and high-carb diets. This is how desires may impact your health:

1. **Nutritional Imbalance:** Foods heavy in sugar, bad fats, and processed carbs are often consumed as a result of cravings. Your diet may become unbalanced due to the absence of vital elements such as vitamins, minerals, and fiber in these meals. This imbalance has the potential to cause inadequacies, weight gain, and health issues in the long run.

2. **Blood Sugar Fluctuations:** Sugar cravings have the potential to send blood sugar levels skyrocketing. Your body produces insulin in response to eating high-sugar meals, which aids in the uptake of glucose by cells. These swings may cause weariness, mood changes, irritation, and desire for more sugar, creating a vicious cycle. This abrupt surge in blood sugar is followed by a swift decrease, resulting in a "sugar crash."

3. **Energy Instability**: When you indulge in high-sugar meals due to cravings, your energy levels may be affected. Although eating sugary snacks could provide you with a quick energy boost, this effect is often fleeting and is followed by a collapse. You experience a rollercoaster effect that leaves you exhausted, drained, and unable to maintain your energy levels throughout the day.

4. **Difficulties with Weight Management:** Food cravings may undermine attempts to control weight by causing overeating. Overindulging in sugary, high-calorie snacks raises the risk of obesity-related health problems including diabetes, heart disease, and joint troubles as well as causes weight gain.

5. **Impact on Mental Health:** Emotional and mental health may be impacted by cravings. The vicious cycle

of desiring, giving in, and then feeling bad or unsatisfied may cause tension, anxiety, and a bad connection with food. Craving-driven emotional eating may exacerbate the issue by becoming a coping method for handling stress or unpleasant feelings.

6. **Nutritional Deficiency:** Recurrent food cravings might be a sign of an underlying nutritional deficiency. For instance, a requirement for chromium, magnesium, or B vitamins may be indicated by a desire for sweets. Ignoring these nutritional requirements over time may result in several health problems.

7. **Long-Term Health Risks:** Consuming unhealthy foods and giving in to persistent cravings may lead to the development of diabetes, insulin resistance, metabolic disorders, cardiovascular diseases, and other illnesses. Making dietary adjustments

and addressing cravings are crucial steps in reducing these long-term health hazards.

In conclusion, unhealthy food cravings may throw off your nutritional balance, cause blood sugar swings and energy instability, make it difficult to maintain a healthy weight, hurt your mental health, and raise your chance of developing long-term health problems. Achieving optimum well-being and energy levels requires understanding the influence of cravings on your health and developing effective techniques to control them.

CHAPTER 2

COMPREHENDING BLOOD SUGAR

Blood glucose, or blood sugar, is the term used to describe the quantity of glucose that is in your bloodstream at any one moment. Simple sugars like glucose are your body's main energy source for cells, particularly those in your muscles and brain. Comprehending blood sugar levels is crucial for preserving general health and wellness. Here are important things to think about:

1. **Regulation:** In non-diabetic people, blood sugar levels normally vary from 70 to 140 milligrams per deciliter (mg/dL). Your body closely monitors blood sugar levels to make sure they remain within this range. The pancreas

secretes the hormone insulin, which is essential for this control. Insulin assists in moving glucose from the circulation into cells for use as fuel or storage when blood sugar levels increase (postprandial).

2. **Glucose Sources:** The meals you consume, particularly carbs, provide you with glucose. During digestion, glucose is produced from carbohydrates and taken into the circulation. While complex carbs, which are found in whole grains, fruits, and vegetables, are digested more slowly and cause blood sugar levels to increase gradually, simple carbohydrates, like sugars and refined grains, cause quick rises in blood sugar levels.

3. **Homeostasis:** Sustaining blood sugar balance is essential for general well-being. Hyperglycemia, or abnormally high blood sugar, may harm organs, blood vessels, and nerves over

time and result in consequences including diabetes, heart disease, renal disease, and eye issues. Conversely, hypoglycemia, or persistently low blood sugar, may result in weakness, disorientation, lightheadedness, and, in extreme situations, unconsciousness.

4. **Monitoring:** Blood sugar levels should be regularly checked, particularly for those who already have diabetes or are at risk of getting it. Frequent blood glucose testing aids in monitoring variations, evaluating the efficacy of treatment, and assisting with educated choices about medicine, nutrition, exercise, and insulin therapy.

5. **Variables Affecting Blood Sugar:** Several variables, such as the following, may affect blood sugar levels:
- Diet: Blood sugar is influenced by the kinds and amounts of lipids, proteins, carbs, and fiber in your diet.

- Physical Activity: Exercise increases insulin sensitivity and the muscles' ability to absorb glucose, which lowers blood sugar levels.
- Stress: Stress hormones can temporarily elevate blood sugar levels by raising them.
- Medication: Several drugs, including several antidepressants and corticosteroids, may alter blood sugar levels.
- Health Conditions: Blood sugar management may be impacted by diseases of the liver or kidneys, diabetes, insulin resistance, and hormonal abnormalities.

6. **Target Levels:** Individual characteristics, age, health, and objectives for managing diabetes all influence target blood sugar levels. For the best blood sugar control, collaborating with healthcare professionals to create individualized

goals and an all-encompassing management strategy is essential.

In conclusion, sustaining optimum health and avoiding issues related to imbalances need an awareness of blood sugar management, sources, monitoring, and the variables that influence it. Maintaining blood sugar homeostasis and general well-being may be facilitated by leading a healthy lifestyle that includes regular exercise, a balanced diet, stress reduction, and frequent monitoring.

An explanation of blood sugar and how it is controlled

The amount of glucose in the circulation is referred to as blood sugar, often called blood glucose. Simple sugars like glucose are the body's main source of energy for cells, especially those in the brain, muscles, and other essential organs. Maintaining ideal health and well-being requires an understanding of blood sugar management.

1. **Glucose Sources:**
Dietary Intake: The main way that glucose enters the circulation is via the breakdown and absorption of dietary carbs. During digestion, carbohydrates are converted to glucose, which is then taken up by the small intestine and into circulation.
- **Glycogen Storage:** Extra glucose is stored in the muscles and liver as glycogen. To keep blood sugar levels steady when they fall (as they do during fasting or in between meals), glycogen is converted into glucose and delivered into the circulation.
Gluconeogenesis: The body may create glucose from non-carbohydrate sources, such as amino acids (from protein) and glycerol (from lipids), via a process known as gluconeogenesis under certain conditions, such as

extended fasting or low carbohydrate consumption.

2. **Controlling Blood Sugar:**
- **Pancreatic Hormones:** Insulin and glucagon, two important hormones secreted by the pancreas, are crucial in controlling blood sugar levels.
Insulin: Released postprandially in response to rising blood sugar levels after meals, insulin is secreted by beta cells in the pancreas. Insulin induces the liver and muscles to store extra glucose as glycogen, hinders the liver's ability to produce new glucose, and helps cells absorb glucose.
- **Glucagon:** When blood sugar levels fall (during fasting or in between meals), the pancreatic alpha cells secrete glucagon. To sustain the supply of energy, glucagon increases blood sugar levels by stimulating the liver's process of converting glycogen to glucose (glycogenolysis) and encouraging gluconeogenesis.

3. **The function of glucagon and insulin:**
Actions of Insulin:
- Promotes the absorption of glucose by cells, especially fat and muscle cells. Encourages the transformation of glucose into glycogen, which is then stored in the muscles and liver.
- Prevents glycogenolysis, the process by which stored glycogen is broken down into glucose.
- Suppresses the synthesis of glucose from sources other than carbohydrates, or gluconeogenesis.
- The Actions of Glucagon:
- Promotes the liver's process of converting glycogen stores into glucose, known as glycogenolysis. Encourages the synthesis of fresh glucose from glycerol and amino acids, a process known as gluconeogenesis.
- Increases blood sugar in response to energy needs, particularly during fasting or physical activity.

4. **Reporting Systems:**
- **Negative Feedback:** A negative feedback loop is involved in blood sugar management. Insulin is produced after a meal to reduce blood sugar when levels increase. On the other hand, glucagon is produced to increase blood sugar levels when they fall.
Feedback Sensors: The pancreas and other organs include specialized cells that monitor blood sugar levels and modify hormone output appropriately. For instance, alpha cells detect low glucose levels and produce glucagon, while beta cells sense high glucose levels and release insulin.

5. **Influential Factors on Blood Sugar Regulation:**
- **Diet:** The kind and amount of lipids, proteins, carbs, and fiber in your diet have an impact on blood sugar levels.

- **Physical Activity:** Exercise helps control blood sugar levels, improves muscle absorption of glucose, and raises insulin sensitivity.
- **Stress:** Hormones related to stress might affect how blood sugar is regulated, causing brief spikes or swings.

Drugs and Health problems: Blood sugar control may be affected by some drugs, health problems (including diabetes), and hormonal imbalances, all of which need to be managed.

All things considered, the pancreas, insulin, glucagon, glycogen storage, and feedback mechanisms are involved in the intricate process of controlling blood sugar. Blood sugar homeostasis is essential for cellular activity, energy production, and general health. People may promote optimum blood sugar management and well-being by making educated lifestyle choices based on their knowledge of the processes governing blood sugar regulation.

Effects of Blood Sugar Levels: High and Low

Hyperglycemia and hypoglycemia, the terms for high and low blood sugar, respectively, may have a serious impact on one's health and general well-being. It is essential to comprehend these impacts to appropriately manage blood sugar levels. The following are the effects of both high and low blood sugar:

Hyperglycemia, or high blood sugar, effects:

1. **Increased Thirst and Urination:** As the body attempts to eliminate extra glucose through urine, high blood sugar levels can cause excessive thirst (polydipsia) and frequent urination (polyuria).

2. **Weakness and Fatigue:** Because cells cannot efficiently absorb glucose for energy production, hyperglycemia can result in feelings of weakness, lethargy, and exhaustion.

3. **Blurry Vision:** Transient blurred vision may result from elevated blood sugar levels affecting the fluid balance in the eyes.

4. **Dry Skin and Mouth:** Increasing urination may cause dehydration, which can result in dry skin and mouth.

5. **Weight Loss:** Because the body cannot properly use glucose for energy, persistent hyperglycemia can lead to weight loss even in the presence of increased appetite.

6. **Increased Risk of Infections:** Because high blood sugar reduces immunity, it increases the risk of

infections, especially those that affect the skin, gums, and urinary tract.

7. **Nerve Damage (Neuropathy): Prolonged hyperglycemia may harm nerves in various parts of the body, causing pain, tingling, and numbness, particularly in the extremities.

8. **Cardiovascular Complications:** Long-term elevated blood sugar levels raise the risk of atherosclerosis, hypertension, heart attacks, and strokes, among other cardiovascular disorders.

Repercussions of Hypoglycemia, or Low Blood Sugar:

1. **Shakiness and Tremors:** Hypoglycemia may result in tremors, shakiness, and a jittery or anxious sensation.

2. **Sweating:** One of the most typical signs of low blood sugar is excessive perspiration or diaphoresis.

3. **Fatigue and Weakness:** Hypoglycemia may cause weariness, weakness, and low energy.

4. **Hunger:** To swiftly boost blood sugar levels, low blood sugar causes hunger and desire for carbs.

5. **Irritability and Confusion:** Hypoglycemia may lead to irritability, mood fluctuations, trouble focusing, and confusion.

6. **Headache:** Some people report having headaches or migraines when their blood sugar is low.

7. **Blurred eyesight:** Hypoglycemia may cause alterations in eyesight, including double or blurred vision.

8. **Severe Symptoms:** If severe hypoglycemia is not treated right away, it may result in seizures, unconsciousness, and coma.

Blood sugar levels should be carefully monitored since they may have major health effects from both high and low levels. To avoid problems and enhance general health, people with diabetes must maintain balanced blood sugar levels via food, medication, routine monitoring, and lifestyle changes.

CHAPTER 3

CAUSES OF BLOOD SUGAR IMBALANCE

Blood sugar abnormalities, which are defined as high (hyperglycemia) or low (hypoglycemia), may be caused by a variety of reasons. Understanding the origins of these imbalances is critical for successful blood sugar management. Here are the main reasons for blood sugar imbalances:

The causes of hyperglycemia (high blood sugar) are:

1. **Unhealthy Diet:** Consuming too many sugary foods, refined carbs, and high-calorie meals may cause blood sugar spikes, which contribute to hyperglycemia.

2. **Insulin Resistance:** Insulin resistance develops when cells lose

responsiveness to insulin, resulting in high blood sugar levels. It is a typical characteristic of type 2 diabetes and metabolic syndrome.

3. **Diabetes:** People with diabetes, both type 1 and type 2, have hyperglycemia because of inadequate insulin production (type 1) or poor insulin action (type 2).

4. **Stress:** Stress hormones like cortisol and adrenaline may elevate blood sugar levels by stimulating gluconeogenesis (the creation of glucose from non-carbohydrate sources) and decreasing insulin sensitivity.

5. **Lack of Physical Activity:** Sedentary lifestyles promote insulin resistance and lower glucose absorption by muscles, resulting in increased blood sugar levels.

6. **Drugs:** Certain drugs, such as corticosteroids, diuretics, and certain antipsychotics, may cause blood sugar to rise as a side effect.

7. **Hormonal Imbalances:** Hormonal diseases such as Cushing's syndrome (excess cortisol), acromegaly (excess growth hormone), and hyperthyroidism may result in hyperglycemia.

8. **Illness or Infection:** Infections, especially those accompanied by inflammation and stress on the body, may cause transient blood sugar spikes.

The causes of hypoglycemia (low blood sugar) are:

1. **drugs:** Certain diabetic drugs, such as insulin and sulfonylureas, may

cause excessive blood sugar drops, resulting in hypoglycemia if not used correctly.

2. **Delayed or Missed Meals:** Skipping or postponing meals for a lengthy period might cause a decline in blood sugar levels, particularly if you are using blood-sugar-lowering drugs.

3. **Excessive Exercise:** Excessive or prolonged physical exercise without enough carbohydrate consumption might deplete glycogen reserves and reduce blood sugar levels.

4. **Alcohol Consumption:** Alcohol may interfere with liver function and inhibit gluconeogenesis, resulting in hypoglycemia, especially in diabetics.

5. **Insulinoma:** An insulinoma is a rare pancreatic tumor that may produce too much insulin, resulting in recurrent hypoglycemia.

6. **Liver or Kidney Disorders:** Liver or kidney illness might impair glucose metabolism, resulting in blood sugar imbalance.

7. **Hormonal Deficiencies:** Hormonal deficiencies, such as cortisol, glucagon, or growth hormone, may lead to hypoglycemia.

8. **Inborn Metabolic Errors:** Rare hereditary disorders that impair enzymes involved in glucose metabolism might result in hypoglycemia.

Managing blood sugar abnormalities requires recognizing and resolving the underlying reasons. Blood sugar control for diabetics requires frequent monitoring, medication adherence, good dietary habits, physical exercise, stress management, and medical supervision.

Dietary Factors and Blood Sugar Imbalances: Sugar Intake and Refined Carbs

Diet plays an important part in blood sugar management, and some dietary components, such as sugar consumption and refined carbs, may have a considerable influence on blood sugar. Understanding how these food components influence glucose metabolism is critical for controlling blood sugar levels. Here's a thorough look at sugar consumption, refined carbs, and their effects on blood sugar:

1. **Sugar intake:**
- **Sources of Sugar:** Sugar may be found in a variety of meals and beverages, including sugary drinks, candies, desserts, processed snacks, and even supposedly healthful items such as flavored yogurts and cereals.
- **Effect on Blood Sugar:** Consuming high-sugar meals causes fast jumps in

blood sugar levels, particularly if they lack fiber or protein to decrease glucose absorption. This increase causes insulin to be released, which helps cells absorb glucose for energy or storage.
- **Insulin Response:** Consuming sugary meals regularly may lead to insulin resistance, which occurs when cells become less sensitive to insulin, resulting in raised blood sugar levels (hyperglycemia) and an increased risk of type 2 diabetes.
- **Empty Calories:** Sugary meals often include empty calories with no nutritious value, which contributes to weight gain, obesity, and other health issues.
- **Desires and Overeating:** Consuming too much sugar may trigger desires for additional sugary foods, perpetuating a cycle of overeating, blood sugar rises, and subsequent falls.

2. **Refined carbohydrates:**

- **Definition:** Refined carbohydrates are processed grains that have had their fiber, vitamins, and minerals removed during refining, leaving mostly starch.
- **Sources:** Common refined carbohydrate sources include white bread, white rice, pasta, pastries, sugary cereals, and white flour-based baked products.
- **Effect on Blood Sugar:** Refined carbs are easily digested and turned into glucose, resulting in fast blood sugar rises comparable to sugar consumption.
- **Insulin Response:** Refined carbs, like sugar, cause an insulin response to control blood sugar levels, but the absence of fiber delays digestion, resulting in a more significant blood sugar surge.
- **Nutritional Deficiency:** Relying extensively on refined carbs may lead to nutritional deficits since they lack the vitamins, minerals, and fiber present in whole grains.

- **Weight Gain and Health Risks:** Regular intake of refined carbs has been linked to weight gain, obesity, insulin resistance, type 2 diabetes, cardiovascular disease, and metabolic syndrome.

Sugar and refined carbohydrate consumption must be managed carefully to maintain balanced blood sugar levels and general health. Strategies for minimizing the influence of these dietary components include:

- **Choosing Whole meals:** Choose whole, unprocessed meals like whole grains, fruits, vegetables, lean meats, and healthy fats to acquire important nutrients and fiber while keeping blood sugar levels stable.
- **Limiting Added Sugars:** Read food labels and restrict meals and drinks containing added sugar. If required, use natural sweeteners such as stevia, monk

fruit, or tiny quantities of honey or maple syrup.
- **Balancing Meals:** Include a variety of carbs, proteins, and fats in your meals to delay digestion, regulate blood sugar levels, and encourage satiety.
- **Favoring Complex Carbohydrates:** Choose complex carbohydrates such as whole grains (e.g., brown rice, quinoa, whole wheat), legumes, and starchy vegetables over refined carbs for longer-lasting energy and improved blood sugar management.
- **Moderation:** Consume sweet snacks and refined carbs in moderation, emphasizing portion management and attentive eating practices.

Individuals may increase general well-being by limiting sugar consumption and eating complete, nutrient-dense meals.

Stress and lack of exercise are two lifestyle factors that might contribute to blood sugar imbalances.

In addition to food considerations, lifestyle decisions like stress management and physical exercise have a substantial impact on blood sugar control. Understanding how these lifestyle variables affect glucose metabolism is critical to maintaining stable blood sugar levels. Here's an in-depth look at stress, lack of exercise, and their effects on blood sugar.

1. **Stress:**
- **Stress Response:** When you are stressed, either physically or emotionally, your body produces stress chemicals such as cortisol and adrenaline. These hormones cause a series of physiological reactions, including the release of glucose into the circulation to give immediate energy (fight-or-flight response).

- **Blood Sugar Spikes:** Chronic or chronic stress may cause repeated spikes in blood sugar levels as glucose is continuously released into the system. This may lead to insulin resistance and higher blood sugar levels over time.
- **Emotional Eating:** Stress may impact eating habits, causing emotional eating and cravings for high-sugar or high-calorie comfort foods, exacerbating blood sugar imbalances.
- **Impact on Insulin Sensitivity:** High cortisol and adrenaline levels may impair insulin sensitivity, making it difficult for cells to react to insulin and properly manage blood sugar.
- **Stress Management Strategies:** Managing stress using relaxation methods, mindfulness practices, regular physical exercise, appropriate sleep, social support, and seeking professional assistance when necessary will help lessen its influence on blood sugar levels.

2. **Lack of exercise:**
- **Insulin Sensitivity:** Regular physical activity, particularly cardiovascular exercise such as walking, running, cycling, or swimming, increases insulin sensitivity and allows cells to absorb glucose more efficiently, resulting in improved blood sugar management.
- **Glucose Utilization:** When exercising, muscles consume glucose for energy, which helps to reduce blood sugar levels. This impact may extend many hours after exercise, boosting total glucose metabolism.
- **Weight control:** Exercise is essential for weight control and obesity prevention, both of which are important variables in maintaining stable blood sugar levels.
- **Stress Reduction:** Physical exercise boosts the release of endorphins (feel-good hormones), which improves mood and lowers blood sugar levels.

- **Consistency is Key:** Consistent and frequent exercise is critical for long-term blood sugar control. Aim for at least 150 minutes of moderate-intensity aerobic activity every week, spaced out across the week.

Combining stress-management strategies with regular physical exercise is an effective way to maintain stable blood sugar levels and general health. Adopting a healthy lifestyle that includes nutritious eating habits, adequate sleep, stress reduction strategies, regular exercise, and medical monitoring (particularly for diabetics) can help optimize glucose metabolism and lower the risk of blood sugar imbalances and related health complications.

Diabetes and insulin resistance are two medical conditions that may cause blood sugar imbalances.

Medical disorders like diabetes and insulin resistance have a significant influence on blood sugar management. Understanding these situations and their impact on glucose metabolism is critical for successfully controlling blood sugar abnormalities. Here's an in-depth look at diabetes, insulin resistance, and its effects on blood sugar:

1. **Diabetes:**
- **Types Of Diabetes:**
- **Type 1 Diabetes:** In type 1 diabetes, the immune system misidentifies and kills insulin-producing beta cells in the pancreas. This results in inadequate insulin synthesis, necessitating ongoing insulin treatment for glucose management.
- **Type 2 Diabetes:** Type 2 diabetes is distinguished by insulin resistance, a condition in which cells become less receptive to insulin. Initially, the pancreas adjusts by making more insulin, but insulin production may

eventually drop, resulting in high blood sugar levels.
- **Effects on Blood Sugar:** Both kinds of diabetes cause high blood sugar levels (hyperglycemia) owing to either inadequate insulin (type 1) or poor insulin action (type 2).
- **Symptoms:** Common symptoms of diabetes include excessive thirst (polydipsia), frequent urination (polyuria), exhaustion, impaired eyesight, sluggish wound healing, and unexplained weight loss.
- **treatment:** Diabetes treatment includes blood sugar monitoring, medication (insulin or oral drugs), dietary changes (carbohydrate counting, glycemic control), regular exercise, stress management, and medical supervision to avoid complications.

2. **Insulin resistance:**
- **Definition:** Insulin resistance develops when cells, notably muscle, fat, and liver cells, become less sensitive to

insulin signals, resulting in reduced glucose absorption.

- **Causes:** Insulin resistance may be caused by genetics, obesity, a sedentary lifestyle, poor eating habits (high sugar and refined carbohydrate consumption), hormonal imbalances, and certain medical diseases.

- **Effects on Blood Sugar:** Insulin resistance causes high blood sugar levels because cells fail to absorb glucose effectively, forcing the pancreas to create more insulin to compensate.

Obesity, physical inactivity, a family history of diabetes, gestational diabetes, polycystic ovarian syndrome (PCOS), and specific ethnicities (such as South Asians, Hispanics, and Native Americans) are all risk factors for insulin resistance.

- **Management:** Managing insulin resistance requires lifestyle modifications such as weight loss, regular physical exercise, appropriate eating habits (low glycemic index foods, fiber-rich meals), stress reduction, enough sleep, and (in certain situations) medication to enhance insulin sensitivity.

Both diabetes and insulin resistance may cause blood sugar abnormalities, such as hyperglycemia (high blood sugar) and hypoglycemia (low blood sugar). Proper management, which includes lifestyle changes, medication adherence, frequent monitoring, and medical supervision, is essential for improving blood sugar control, avoiding problems, and boosting overall health and well-being.

CCHAPTER 4

GLUCOSE-HEALTHY DIET

A glucose-healthy diet focuses on maintaining stable blood sugar levels, which promotes general health and well-being. This sort of diet is very good for those with diabetes, insulin resistance, or who want to avoid blood sugar abnormalities. Here are the main concepts and components of a glucose-healthy diet:

1. **The emphasis is on whole foods:**
- Include a wide range of entire, unprocessed foods, such as fruits, vegetables, whole grains, legumes, nuts, seeds, lean proteins, and healthy fats.
- Whole foods are high in important nutrients, fiber, antioxidants, and phytonutrients, which help regulate blood sugar and promote general health.

2. **Foods With a Low Glycemic Index (GI)**
- Choose foods with a low glycemic index, which indicates they have a slower and more consistent effect on blood sugar levels.
Low GI foods include non-starchy vegetables (e.g., leafy greens, broccoli, cauliflower), whole grains (e.g., quinoa, barley, oats), legumes (e.g., lentils, chickpeas, beans), and most fruits (e.g., berries, apples, citrus fruits).

3. **balanced macronutrients:**
- Include a variety of carbs, proteins, and fats in your meals to increase satiety, delay digestion, and regulate blood sugar levels.
- To minimize high blood sugar spikes, choose complex carbs (whole grains, veggies, fruits) over refined carbohydrates (sugary meals, white bread, and pastries).

4. **Healthy fats:**

- Consume healthy fats in moderation, such as avocados, nuts, seeds, olive oil, and fatty fish (e.g., salmon, mackerel). When ingested as part of a well-balanced diet, healthy fats promote heart health, give long-lasting energy, and aid in blood sugar regulation.

5. **Portion Control**
- Pay attention to portion sizes to prevent overeating and blood sugar rises.
To maintain a healthy weight and blood sugar management, use smaller plates, measure portion sizes, and keep track of your calorie consumption.

6. **Limit added sugars and refined carbs:**
- Limit your intake of meals and beverages with added sugars, such as sugary drinks, candy, desserts, and processed snacks.
- Limit your consumption of refined carbs such as white bread, rice, pasta,

and pastries, which may trigger fast blood sugar changes.

7. **Fiber-rich foods:**
- Eat fiber-rich foods including whole grains, vegetables, fruits, legumes, and nuts to enhance digestive health, decrease carbohydrate absorption, and regulate blood sugar levels.
- Consume at least 25-30 grams of fiber every day from dietary sources.

8. **Hydration:**
- Stay hydrated by drinking lots of water all day. Avoid sugary drinks and instead drink water, herbal teas, or infused water.

9. **Meal planning and timing:**
- Eat balanced meals and snacks that include carbs, proteins, and fats to avoid blood sugar spikes and crashes.
- Maintain stable blood sugar levels by eating at regular intervals and spacing meals equally throughout the day.

10. **Regular physical activity:**
- Incorporate regular physical activity into your regimen, since it improves insulin sensitivity, stimulates glucose absorption by muscles, and helps with overall blood sugar management.
- Before beginning any new workout regimen, consult with a healthcare practitioner, particularly if you have any pre-existing health concerns.

Individuals who follow a glucose-healthy diet that emphasizes whole foods, low GI options, balanced macronutrients, portion control, and regular physical activity can support optimal blood sugar regulation, reduce the risk of blood sugar imbalances and related health issues, and promote overall well-being. Consulting with a licensed dietician or healthcare practitioner may give tailored advice and assistance for good blood sugar management.

The significance of balanced meals including complex carbohydrates, proteins, and healthy fats

Balanced meals with a variety of complex carbs, proteins, and healthy fats are essential for maintaining stable blood sugar levels, supporting general health, and giving sustained energy throughout the day. Here's why each of these components is necessary and what foods to include in a balanced meal:

1. **Complex carbohydrates:**
- **Importance:** Complex carbs provide fiber, vitamins, minerals, and antioxidants. They have a delayed influence on blood sugar levels than simple carbs, resulting in prolonged energy and satiety.
- **Foods To Include:**
- veggies: Include a range of colorful veggies such as spinach, broccoli, cauliflower, bell peppers, carrots, and zucchini. These are low in calories yet

abundant in fiber, vitamins, and antioxidants.

- Whole Grains: Choose whole grains such as brown rice, quinoa, barley, oats, whole wheat pasta, and whole grain bread. Compared to refined grains, they have more fiber, complex carbs, and minerals.

- Legumes include lentils, chickpeas, black beans, kidney beans, and peas. They provide an abundance of plant-based protein, fiber, and carbs.

2. **Proteins:**
- **Importance:** Proteins are necessary for tissue growth and repair, immune function support, and muscle mass maintenance. Including protein in meals helps to regulate blood sugar levels, improve fullness, and avoid overeating.
- **Foods To Include:**
- Lean Proteins: Consume skinless poultry, fish (salmon, tuna, trout), tofu, tempeh, lean cuts of beef or pig, eggs,

and low-fat dairy products such as Greek yogurt or cottage cheese.
- Plant-Based Proteins: Include plant-based proteins such as beans, lentils, chickpeas, edamame, quinoa, nuts, seeds, and soybean products. These include a range of nutrients and are lower in saturated fat than certain animal-based proteins.

3. **Healthy fats:**
- **Importance:** Healthy fats are required for brain function, hormone synthesis, and fat-soluble vitamin absorption (A, D, E, K). Including healthy fats in meals slows digestion, regulates blood sugar levels, and promotes satiety.
- **Foods To Include:**
- Avocados: Slices of avocado may be added to salads, sandwiches, or smoothies to provide healthful monounsaturated fats, fiber, and vitamins.

- Nuts and Seeds: Use almonds, walnuts, chia seeds, flaxseeds, pumpkin seeds, and sunflower seeds as toppings for yogurt, cereal, and salads. These are high in omega-3 fatty acids and provide crispness to dishes.
- Olive Oil: Use extra virgin olive oil while cooking or pouring over salads. It includes both monounsaturated fats and antioxidants.
- Fatty Fish: Eat oily fish like salmon, mackerel, sardines, and trout at least twice a week to get omega-3 fatty acids, which help with heart health and inflammation.

Individuals may enjoy a nutrient-rich diet by including a range of vegetables, whole grains, lean meats, and healthy fats in balanced meals. This diet promotes satiety, supports appropriate blood sugar regulation, and adds to general health and well-being. Incorporating these items into meal plans and selecting whole, less processed choices wherever feasible will help you live a healthier lifestyle.

Avoid or limit the following foods for blood sugar management:

1. **Sugary Snacks & Sweets:**
- **Avoidance:** Limit or avoid items rich in added sugars, including sweets, chocolates, pastries, cookies, cakes, ice cream, sugary cereals, and sweetened beverages (sodas, fruit juices, energy drinks).
- **Reason:** The high sugar content of these meals may produce fast increases in blood sugar levels, resulting in imbalances and an increased risk of insulin resistance, diabetes, weight gain, and other health concerns.

2. **Processed Foods With Added Sugar:**
- **Limitation:** Avoid processed foods with added sugars, such as morning cereals, flavored yogurts, granola bars,

sauces, dressings, and packaged snacks (chips, crackers, baked goods).
- **Reason:** Processed foods often include hidden sugars and bad fats, which may lead to blood sugar imbalances, inflammation, and metabolic issues. When feasible, choose whole foods that have been lightly processed.

3. **Refined carbohydrates:**
- **Avoidance/Limitation:** Limit your consumption of refined carbs including white bread, white rice, pasta made with refined flour, sugary cereals, and pastries.
- **Reason:** Refined carbs have a high glycemic index, resulting in rapid blood sugar fluctuations. They lack the fiber and minerals present in whole grains, which may lead to insulin resistance, weight gain, and metabolic problems.

4. **Sugary beverages:**

- **Avoidance:** Stay away from sugary beverages such as soda, sweetened iced tea, energy drinks, fruit punches, and sugary coffee drinks.
- **Reason:** These beverages are high in added sugars and empty calories, which causes rapid blood sugar spikes and promotes harmful weight gain, dental difficulties, and metabolic illnesses.

5. **Highly processed and fried food:**
- **Limitation:** Reduce your intake of highly processed foods such as fast food, deep-fried snacks (fries, chips), processed meats (sausages, hot dogs), and pre-packaged meals.
- **Reason:** These foods often include harmful fats, salt, additives, and preservatives, which contribute to inflammation, insulin resistance, weight gain, and cardiovascular risks.

6. **Artificial sweeteners:**

- **Moderation:** Use artificial sweeteners such as aspartame, sucralose, and saccharin sparingly, if at all.
- **Reason:** Although artificial sweeteners deliver sweetness without calories, some research suggests that they may still have an impact on blood sugar levels, gut bacteria, and appetite control. When appropriate, use natural sweeteners such as stevia or monk fruit.

7. **Alcohol:**
- **Moderation:** Drink alcohol in moderation and be aware of its effect on blood glucose levels.
- **Reason:** Alcohol may impair liver function, glucose metabolism, and insulin sensitivity, causing variations in blood sugar levels. Limit your alcohol consumption and select low-sugar beverages such as dry wines or light beers.

By avoiding or restricting certain items in your diet and concentrating on full, nutrient-dense choices, you may improve blood sugar control, lower your risk of blood sugar imbalances and associated health problems, promote overall well-being, and live a healthier lifestyle. To achieve optimum blood sugar management, practice mindful eating, read food labels, and emphasize whole foods.

CHAPTER 5

MANAGING CRAVINGS

Managing cravings is a crucial part of keeping blood sugar levels stable and general wellness. Cravings for sugary, high-carb, or unhealthy meals may cause blood sugar imbalances, weight gain, and other health problems. Here are practical ways to manage cravings:

1. **Eat Regular and Balanced Meals:**
- Prepare and eat nutritious meals that contain complex carbs, lean proteins, healthy fats, and fiber-rich foods.
- Eating frequent meals throughout the day helps to maintain blood sugar levels and minimizes the probability of severe cravings.

2. **Combine Protein and Healthy Fats:**

- Include protein-rich foods and healthy fats in your meals and snacks to increase satiety and reduce blood sugar swings.
- Protein sources include lean meats, fish, eggs, beans, tofu, and nuts. Avocados, olive oil, nuts, seeds, and fatty seafood are all sources of healthy fats.

3. **Select Low-Glycemic Foods:**
- Choose low-glycemic index (GI) foods, which have a slower influence on blood sugar levels, reducing cravings and maintaining energy levels.
- Low-GI foods include non-starchy vegetables, whole grains, legumes, and most fruits (particularly berries).

4. **Stay hydrated:**
- Drink plenty of water throughout the day to keep hydrated and lessen sensations of hunger or cravings, since thirst is frequently confused with hunger.

5. **Try Mindful Eating:**
- Pay attention to your hunger and fullness signals, and engage in mindful eating by concentrating on the tastes, textures, and feelings of each mouthful.
- Avoid distractions when eating, such as watching television or using electronic gadgets, since these may lead to thoughtless overeating.

6. **Addressing Emotional Triggers:**
- Recognize and address emotional factors that might cause cravings, such as stress, boredom, loneliness, or worry.
- Look for alternate methods to deal with emotions, such as practicing relaxation techniques, participating in hobbies, socializing, or obtaining help from friends or a therapist.

7. **Plan for Healthy Snacks:**
- Make healthful snacks easily accessible to fulfill desires without jeopardizing blood sugar management. Examples include Greek yogurt with berries, a tiny handful of almonds, carrot sticks with hummus, and apple slices with almond butter.

8. **Getting Adequate Sleep:**
- Aim for 7-9 hours of excellent sleep every night, since insufficient sleep disrupts hunger hormones and increases cravings for high-calorie meals.

9. **Exercise regularly:**
- Engage in regular physical activity, since it helps control hunger, boost mood, decrease stress, and improve overall health.

- Incorporate activities that you love into your regimen, such as walking, dancing, yoga, or strength training.

10. **Practice moderation:**
- Allow yourself to enjoy occasional delights or indulgences in moderation, guilt-free. Depriving oneself totally might cause emotions of deprivation and even binge eating episodes.

By combining these tactics into your daily routine, you may successfully control cravings, maintain stable blood sugar levels, and foster a healthy relationship with food. Remember that consistency and conscious decisions are essential for long-term success in controlling cravings and sustaining overall health.

- Recognizing the reasons behind cravings (emotions, behaviors)

Cravings are often caused by a mix of emotional and behavioral tendencies. Understanding these triggers allows people to establish successful desire management techniques.

Here's an investigation of the common causes of cravings:

1. **Emotional triggers:**
- **Stress:** Stress is a key emotional trigger for cravings. During stressful conditions, the body produces chemicals such as cortisol and adrenaline, which may stimulate hunger and desire for high-calorie, comforting foods.
- **Boredom:** Feelings of boredom or monotony may lead to thoughtless eating and snack cravings, particularly if food is used to relieve boredom or find excitement.

- **Sorrow or Depression:** Emotional pain, such as sorrow or depression, may cause cravings for foods that bring brief comfort or pleasure, which are often heavy in sugar or fat.
- **Anxiety or anxiety:** Anxiety and anxiety may cause cravings as a coping technique to relieve stress or distract from unpleasant feelings.

2. **Habitual triggers:**
- **Environmental Cues:** Environmental cues like seeing or smelling food, being in certain areas (such as a kitchen or a favorite restaurant), or being in social situations where food is plentiful may cause cravings even when you are not physically hungry.
- **Time of Day:** Certain periods of the day, such as late afternoon or evening, maybe frequent triggers for cravings, particularly if snacking occurs at those times.

- **Routine Behaviors:** Certain activities or routines, such as watching TV, working at a desk, or surfing the internet, might cause cravings because of habit or connection with previous behaviors.
- **Social Influence:** Social circumstances, gatherings, or peer pressure may cause desires for foods or beverages that are often eaten in social contexts.

3. **Physical Trigger:**
- **Hunger:** Physical hunger is a typical cause of cravings. When blood sugar levels drop owing to extended fasting, the body signals hunger, resulting in cravings for rapid energy sources such as sugary foods.
- **Thirst:** Dehydration or insufficient fluid intake might be misinterpreted for hunger, resulting in cravings. Drinking water or other hydrated liquids may help alleviate thirst-related cravings.

- **Nutritional shortages:** Certain vitamin shortages, such as low magnesium levels, might cause cravings for certain foods. A balanced diet with enough nutrition might help alleviate these cravings.

4. **Social and cultural influences:**
- **Societal standards:** Cultural and societal variables, such as food availability, festivities, customs, and eating standards, may all contribute to cravings for certain meals.
- **Marketing and Advertising:** Exposure to marketing, advertising, and media that promote certain foods or drinks might impact desires and food selection.

Managing cravings:
- **Awareness:** Recognize and recognize your desire triggers, whether

they are emotional, habitual, environmental, or social.
- **Mindfulness:** Practice mindfulness practices to become more aware of your craving-related thoughts, emotions, and actions without passing judgment.
- **Emotional Regulation:** Practice healthy coping skills for controlling feelings like tension, boredom, worry, or sorrow, such as deep breathing, meditation, exercise, or participating in pleasant hobbies.
- **Healthy Alternatives:** Keep healthy snacks on hand to satisfy cravings while maintaining blood sugar management. Choose from fruits, veggies, nuts, Greek yogurt, and whole-grain snacks.
- **Divert and Delay:** When a desire comes, divert yourself with a non-food-related activity (for example, going for a walk, listening to music, or contacting a friend) and wait a specific amount of time to see whether it passes.
- **Modify Habits:** Identify and change any habitual actions or routines

that cause cravings. For example, if watching television often leads to eating, look for other hobbies or snacks to break the pattern.
- **Seek Support:** Discuss your objectives and problems with supportive friends, family members, or a healthcare professional who may provide encouragement, accountability, and advice.

Standing and addressing desire triggers allow people to build better habits, regulate emotional eating, and make mindful choices that promote balanced blood sugar levels and general well-being.

- **Strategies for overcoming cravings (mindful eating, distraction strategies).**

1. **Mindful eating:
- **Awareness:** Practice mindful eating by focusing on the sensory experience of eating, such as the taste, texture, scent, and look of foods.
- **Slow Down:** Eat slowly and relish each meal, chewing properly and pausing between bites. This gives your brain time to recognize fullness and contentment.
- **Listen to Your Body:** Pay attention to your body's hunger and fullness signs. Eat when you're physically hungry and stop when you're comfortably full, rather than relying on emotions or external signals.
- **Avoid Distractions:** Limit distractions when eating, such as watching TV, using electronics, or working. Concentrate entirely on the act of eating and enjoying the meal without multitasking.

2. Distraction Techniques:

- **Engage in Activities:** When you have a need, divert yourself by doing something non-food-related that you love. This might involve taking a stroll, engaging in a hobby, reading a book, listening to music, or solving a puzzle.
- **Physical Activity:** Include physical activity in your daily routine since it may help decrease cravings, enhance mood, and promote overall well-being.
- **Deep Breathing:** Use deep breathing exercises or relaxation methods to alleviate stress and cravings. Deep breathing may assist in relaxing the mind and reduce emotional triggers for eating.
- **Phone a Friend:** Contact a sympathetic friend or family member to have a talk or social engagement. Connecting with people might help to distract you from your desires while also providing emotional support.
- **Change Your Environment:** If feasible, alter your surroundings to

eliminate temptations or triggers for cravings.

CHAPTER 6

STRESS-MANAGEMENT STRATEGIES

Stress is a typical occurrence in today's fast-paced society and may have serious consequences for physical, mental, and emotional well-being. Effective stress management practices may assist in mitigating the harmful impacts of stress and enhance overall quality of life. Here are some essential stress-management strategies:

1. **Identify stressors:**
- Recognize and recognize stressors in your life, such as job demands, marital problems, financial difficulties, health worries, or significant life changes.

- Keep a stress diary to capture stress causes, symptoms, and trends so you can better understand your stressors.

2. **Practice Relaxation Techniques:**
- Use relaxation methods to calm your mind and body. Deep breathing techniques, gradual muscular relaxation, guided visualization, meditation, and mindfulness are a few examples.
- Incorporate frequent relaxation sessions into your daily routine to improve calm and lessen stress reactions.

3. **Physical activity:**
- Incorporate regular physical activity into your schedule; exercise is an excellent stress reliever. Choose your favorite activities, such as walking, running, dancing, yoga, or swimming.
- Aim for at least 30 minutes of moderate-intensity exercise most days

of the week to improve your mood, decrease anxiety, and promote relaxation.

4. **Healthy lifestyle habits:**
- Prioritize a well-balanced diet rich in nutrients, appropriate water, and frequent meals to promote general health and stress resistance.
- Get enough sleep every night, aiming for 7-9 hours of quality sleep, since sleep deficiency may worsen stress and decrease coping skills.
- Limit coffee, alcohol, and tobacco usage, since these chemicals may increase tension and anxiety.

5. **Time management:**
- Organize and prioritize chores to better manage time and avoid feelings of overload. Use calendars, planners, to-do lists, and task-prioritizing approaches.

- Divide projects into smaller, more achievable stages to minimize procrastination and stress caused by deadlines.

6. **Set boundaries:**
- Set clear boundaries in your personal and professional lives to safeguard your time, energy, and overall well-being. Learn to say no to excessive obligations or requests that cause stress.
- Communicate assertively and respectfully about your needs and limitations with others.

7. **Social Support:
- Maintain contact with helpful friends, family, and support groups. Talking to people, sharing your experiences, and getting emotional support may all help to decrease stress and offer perspective.
- Seek professional help from a therapist or counselor if pressures are

overpowering or affecting your mental health.

8. **Mindfulness and Mind-Body Practice:**
- Use mindfulness practices to be present in the moment, increase self-awareness, and lessen ruminations about past or future stresses.
- Use mind-body techniques like yoga, tai chi, qigong, or guided visualization to improve relaxation, stress resilience, and emotional balance.

9. **Positive Coping Strategies:**
- Create good coping methods for stress management, such as problem-solving, reframing negative thoughts, practicing gratitude, humor, creativity, or participating in enjoyable hobbies and activities.

- Concentrate on solutions and activities within your power rather than events outside your control.

10. **Get Professional Help:**
- If stress becomes overpowering, chronic, or has a substantial effect on everyday functioning, see a mental health professional. Therapy, counseling, and stress management programs may provide further support and coping methods.

By adopting these stress management techniques into your daily routine, you may successfully decrease stress, boost resilience, improve overall well-being, and negotiate life's obstacles with more ease and balance. Experiment with several strategies to see what works best for you, and then develop a tailored stress management strategy that promotes your health and happiness.

Effect of stress on blood sugar levels.
The Effect of Stress on Blood Sugar Levels

Stress may have a major influence on blood sugar levels, particularly for those who have diabetes, insulin resistance, or are predisposed to blood sugar abnormalities. Here are the main ways that stress influences blood sugar levels:

1. **Hormonal response:**
- When you are stressed, your body produces chemicals like cortisol and adrenaline as part of the "fight or flight" reaction.
- Cortisol stimulates glucose synthesis in the liver and lowers insulin sensitivity in

cells, resulting in elevated blood sugar levels.
- Adrenaline causes the release of stored glucose into the circulation for fast energy, which contributes to high blood sugar levels.

2. **Insulin resistance:**
- Chronic stress and persistently high cortisol levels may lead to insulin resistance, a condition in which cells become less receptive to insulin's effects.
- Insulin resistance limits cells' capacity to absorb glucose from the circulation, resulting in increased blood sugar levels over time.

3. Changes in Eating Patterns:
- Stress may alter eating habits, causing changes in food choices and eating patterns.
- Some people may have stress-related cravings for high-carbohydrate, sugary

meals, which may trigger sudden blood sugar rises.
- Emotional eating or stress eating may lead to overeating and blood sugar swings.

4. Physical inactivity:
- Stress may make people less motivated or unable to participate in regular physical exercise.
Reduced physical activity may have an influence on blood sugar management by lowering muscle glucose absorption and insulin sensitivity.

5. **Sleep Disturbances**
- Chronic stress may cause sleep disruptions including insomnia and poor sleep quality.
- Inadequate sleep may modify hormone levels such as cortisol and growth hormone, affecting blood sugar regulation and insulin sensitivity.

6. **Medical Adherence:**
- Stressful events or periods of severe stress might impair medication adherence in people with diabetes or other blood sugar-related illnesses.
- Failure to take medicine as recommended or to adhere to treatment programs might cause variations in blood sugar levels.

7. **Emotional and Mental Health Impacts:**
- Stress may have a significant influence on emotional and mental health, increasing anxiety, sadness, and mood swings.
- Emotional strain may cause physiological reactions that affect blood sugar levels, such as increased cortisol production and changes in eating habits.

8. **Long-term effects:**
- Chronic stress and persistently raised blood sugar levels may lead to long-term health problems, such as an increased chance of developing type 2 diabetes, cardiovascular disease, and other metabolic diseases.
- Effective stress management is vital for maintaining good blood sugar control and general health.

Managing Stress to Improve Blood Sugar Control:

1. **Stress Reduction Techniques:**
- Use stress-reduction techniques like deep breathing exercises, meditation, mindfulness, yoga, progressive muscle relaxation, or guided imagery to promote relaxation and lower cortisol levels.
- Participate in activities that bring you joy, relaxation, and a sense of calm, such

as spending time in nature, listening to music, pursuing hobbies, or socializing with supportive friends and family.

2. **Regular physical activity:**
- Incorporate regular physical activity into your daily routine, as exercise is a natural stress reliever that also improves insulin sensitivity.
- Select activities that you enjoy, and aim for a mix of aerobic, strength, flexibility, and balance exercises.

3. **Healthy Food Habits:**
- To support stable blood sugar levels, eat a balanced diet rich in nutrients, drink plenty of water, and eat at regular intervals.
- Practice mindful eating, pay attention to hunger cues, and choose nutritious foods to avoid stress-related or emotional eating.

4. **Quality sleep:**
- Prioritize good sleep hygiene habits to improve sleep quality and duration. Establish a relaxing bedtime routine, limit screen time before bed, and create a comfortable sleeping environment.
- Consistent, restful sleep promotes hormone regulation, stress resilience, and overall health.

5. **Seek Support:**
- Consult a healthcare provider, counselor, or mental health professional if you are experiencing chronic stress, anxiety, or difficulty managing stress.
- Join support groups, attend stress management workshops, or take part in stress reduction programs to learn effective coping strategies.

Individuals who address stress and implement healthy coping mechanisms can better manage blood sugar levels, improve insulin sensitivity, and reduce the risk of complications caused by stress-related blood sugar fluctuations. Consistent self-care techniques, lifestyle changes, and getting professional help when necessary are all important components of stress management for good health and wellness.

- Techniques for stress reduction (meditation, deep breathing, yoga)

Techniques to Reduce Stress

Reducing stress is critical for general health and may be accomplished via a variety of relaxation practices that promote tranquility, awareness, and emotional equilibrium. Here are helpful ways to reduce stress:

1. **Meditation:**

- **Mindfulness Meditation:** Focus on the present moment without judgment. Sit comfortably, shut your eyes, and focus on your breathing, physical sensations, thoughts, and emotions. Allow them to come and leave without any attachments.
- **Guided Meditation:** Use guided meditation recordings or apps to walk you through relaxation techniques, visualizations, and mindfulness practices. Follow along with relaxing instructions to relieve stress and improve mental clarity.
- **Transcendental Meditation:** Discover Transcendental Meditation (TM) practices, which include quietly repeating a mantra to calm the mind and achieve profound relaxation. TM is done for 15-20 minutes twice every day.

2. Deep Breathing Exercises:
- **Diaphragmatic Breathing:** Practice diaphragmatic breathing (also known as

belly breathing) by inhaling deeply through your nose and allowing your abdomen to expand before gently expelling through your mouth, letting go of tension. Repeat many times to relax.
- **4-7-8 Breathing:** Practice the 4-7-8 breathing method by inhaling for 4 seconds, holding your breath for 7 seconds, then gently expelling for 8 seconds. This rhythm promotes relaxation and lowers stress reactions.
- **Box Breathing:** Use box breathing methods to inhale for 4 seconds, hold for 4 seconds, exhale for 4 seconds, then pause for 4 seconds before repeating. This rhythmical breathing pattern relaxes the neurological system.

3. **Yoga:**
- **Hatha Yoga:** Engage in mild Hatha yoga positions that emphasize relaxation, stretching, and mindful movement. Use stances like Child's

Pose, Cat-Cow Stretch, Forward Fold, and Legs Up the Wall to relieve tension.
- **Restorative Yoga:** Practice restorative yoga postures using props such as bolsters, blankets, and blocks to promote deep relaxation and tension release. Poses such as Savasana (Corpse Pose), Supported Bridge Pose, and Reclining Bound Angle Pose encourage relaxation.
- **Yoga Nidra:** Practice Yoga Nidra (yogic sleep) to achieve profound relaxation and conscious awareness. Follow guided Yoga Nidra sessions to reduce stress and enhance general health.

4. **Progressive Muscular Relaxation (PMR):**
- Use Progressive Muscle Relaxation (PMR) methods to gradually tense and relax muscle groups in your body. Begin with your toes and work your way up to

your head, concentrating on releasing tension and increasing relaxation.

5. **Visualization and Images:**
- Visualize and imagine tranquil, relaxing sights or situations. Close your eyes, imagine yourself in a peaceful environment (such as a beach, forest, or mountain), and use your senses (sight, sound, and smell) to induce relaxation.

6. **Mindful Practices:**
- Practice everyday mindfulness techniques including mindful walking, mindful eating, and attentive listening. Pay attention to sensations, thoughts, and emotions without passing judgment, developing a feeling of presence and awareness.

7. **Journalism and Expressive Writing:**

- Write in a notebook or practice expressive writing to examine your ideas, feelings, and worries. Writing may be a therapeutic way to process emotions, achieve insight, and release psychological stress.

8. **Nature and outdoor activities:**
- Spend time in nature and participate in outdoor activities that encourage relaxation and connection to the natural environment. Take a stroll through parks, woods, or gardens, try gardening, or engage in outdoor activities.

9. **Laughter Therapy.**
- Incorporate laughter therapy by watching comedies, doing laughter yoga courses, or participating in fun activities that encourage laughter and humor. Laughter releases endorphins, lowers stress hormones, and improves mood.

10. **Social Support and Connections:**
- Seek help from friends, family, or support groups to share your experiences, vent your feelings, and gain empathy and understanding. Social interaction and emotional support are critical for stress management.

11. **Professional support:**
- Seek professional help from a therapist, counselor, or mental health professional if stress becomes overwhelming, chronic, or seriously impairs everyday function. Therapy sessions may help with coping skills, stress management methods, and emotional support.

Incorporating these relaxation methods into your daily routine will help you decrease stress, increase relaxation, improve mental health, and improve your overall quality of life. Experiment with several strategies to see what works best for you, and then develop a tailored stress management strategy that promotes your health and happiness.

- Integrating relaxing techniques into everyday living.
Integrating Relaxation Practices into Everyday Life

Integrating relaxation techniques into your daily routine is critical for stress management, boosting well-being, and living a balanced lifestyle. Making relaxing a regular part of your day may help you decrease stress, increase mental clarity, boost mood, and create a feeling of peace. Here are **Some useful strategies for implementing relaxation methods into your everyday life:**

1. **Morning Routine:**
- Begin the day with a few minutes of deep breathing or mindfulness meditation. Set aside time to concentrate on your breathing, center yourself, and make good plans for the day ahead.
- Warm up your body and encourage relaxation with moderate stretches or yoga positions before beginning your daily routine.

2. **Midday Breaks**
- Take small pauses throughout the day to refuel and unwind. Use these pauses to engage in deep breathing, visualization, or gradual muscular relaxation.
- Take a short meditative stroll to clear your thoughts and lessen tension.

3. **Lunch Time Relaxation:**

- Use your lunch hour to unwind and relax. Savor each mouthful of your food, paying attention to its tastes and sensations.
- Relax by listening to peaceful music, reading a book or inspiring quotations, or engaging in a quick meditation session around lunchtime.

4. **Afternoon refreshment:**
- Incorporate stimulating and calming activities into your afternoon routine. Take a quick power nap if necessary to rejuvenate and increase productivity.
- Try chair yoga or desk stretches to relieve muscular tension and improve posture after sitting for an extended length of time.

5. **Evening Wind Down:**
- Establish a relaxing evening routine to alert your body and mind that it's time to unwind and prepare for sleep. To

limit stimulation, turn off all electronic devices at least one hour before sleep.
- Relaxation methods such as moderate yoga, deep breathing exercises, or guided meditation might help you relax and sleep better.
- Relax and relax by taking a warm bath or shower, listening to calming music, or reading a book.

6. **Bedtime rituals:**
- Create nighttime routines that encourage relaxation and indicate to your body that it is time to rest. While resting in bed, do gradual muscular relaxation or visualization exercises.
To improve sleep quality, provide a pleasant sleep environment that includes subdued lighting, soft bedding, and a cool room temperature.

7. **Mindful Breaks During the Day:**

- Incorporate thoughtful moments into your everyday routine, such as taking a few deep breaths before replying to emails or practicing mindful eating during meals.
- To change your attention away from tension and toward appreciation, practice thankfulness by meditating on pleasant elements of your day or keeping a gratitude notebook.

8. **Consistent Practices:**
- Make relaxation activities a regular part of your daily routine by setting out time for them each day. Set reminders or alarms to encourage you to indulge in relaxing activities.
- Experiment with various relaxation methods to see what works best for you, and include a range of activities into your daily routine to promote overall stress management.

9. **Mindful Technology Usage:**
- Use technology wisely by adding relaxation applications, guided meditation recordings, or relaxing music playlists into your daily routine.
- Set limits on screen use, particularly before bedtime, to encourage relaxation and increase sleep quality.

10. **Flexibility and adaptability:**
- Be flexible and adaptive in your relaxation techniques, modifying them to fit your daily schedule, preferences, and requirements.
- Remember that consistency is essential for enjoying the advantages of relaxation activities, so include self-care and relaxation in your entire health regimen.

By implementing these relaxation techniques into your everyday routine, you may live a more balanced, aware, and stress-resistant existence.

Consistent use of relaxation methods boosts general well-being, improves coping skills, and builds a feeling of serenity in the face of life's adversities. Start small, be gentle with yourself, and gradually establish a pattern that promotes your mental and emotional well-being.

CHAPTER 7.

SLEEP AND BLOOD SUGAR

Sleep and Blood Sugar: Understanding the Connection

The link between sleep and blood sugar levels is complicated and important, with sleep quality and duration influencing glucose metabolism, insulin sensitivity, and overall metabolic health. Here's an outline of how sleep affects blood sugar levels and how to optimize sleep for improved glucose control:

1. **Effects of Sleep on Blood Sugar:**
- Sleep regulates blood sugar levels, insulin secretion, and glucose metabolism. Inadequate or poor-quality sleep may disturb these processes, causing blood sugar abnormalities.
- Inadequate or irregular sleep patterns might reduce insulin sensitivity, raise insulin resistance, and result in

increased fasting blood glucose levels, postprandial (after-meal) spikes, and total glucose fluctuation.

2. **Hormonal regulation:**
- Sleep affects hormone control, including insulin, glucagon, cortisol, growth hormone, leptin, and ghrelin, all of which play important roles in glucose homeostasis, appetite management, energy balance, and metabolic function.
- Inadequate sleep may disturb the balance of these hormones, resulting in dysregulated glucose metabolism, increased appetite, cravings for sweet or high-carbohydrate meals, and trouble controlling blood sugar levels.

3. **The effects of sleep deprivation:**
- Chronic sleep deprivation or poor sleep quality may contribute to insulin resistance, which occurs when cells become less receptive to insulin, resulting in raised blood sugar levels and an increased risk of type 2 diabetes.

- Sleep deprivation may also include increased appetite, changed food choices, decreased physical activity, weariness, mood problems, cognitive impairment, and elevated stress levels, all of which can influence blood sugar regulation.

4. **Tips for Better Sleep and Glucose Control:**
- Create a Consistent Sleep pattern: Aim for a regular sleep pattern by going to bed and getting up at the same time every day, especially on weekends, to regulate circadian rhythms and improve sleep quality.
- Establish a soothing nighttime Routine: Create a soothing nighttime routine that includes activities like reading, having a warm bath, doing deep breathing exercises, or listening to quiet music to signal to your body that it's time to unwind and prepare for sleep.
- Improve Sleep Quality: Create a sleep-friendly atmosphere by keeping

your bedroom dark, quiet, and cool, utilizing comfortable bedding and pillows, decreasing noise and distractions, and limiting computer usage before bedtime.

- Limit Stimulants and coffee: Avoid drinking stimulants like coffee, nicotine, and alcohol close to bedtime since they may interfere with sleep onset, disturb sleep cycles, and lower overall sleep quality.
- Practice Stress Reduction Techniques: To reduce stress, increase relaxation, and enhance sleep quality, try meditation, yoga, progressive muscle relaxation, mindfulness activities, or journaling.
- Use sleep monitoring apps or devices to keep track of your sleep patterns, length, sleep phases, disturbances, and general sleep quality. Reviewing sleep data may help you find areas for

improvement and make changes to your sleeping patterns.

- Address Sleep Disorders: If you have chronic sleep issues, such as snoring, sleep apnea, insomnia, restless legs syndrome, or other sleep disorders, see a healthcare expert for proper management and assistance.

The importance of quality sleep for hyperglycemia regulation.

Quality sleep is critical for glucose control and general metabolic health. Adequate and restorative sleep is required to maintain normal blood sugar levels, insulin sensitivity, and metabolic function. Here are the main reasons why quality sleep is essential for glucose regulation:

1. **Insulin sensitivity:**
- Quality sleep is strongly connected to insulin sensitivity, which refers to how well cells react to insulin's signal to absorb glucose from the circulation.

Adequate sleep promotes insulin sensitivity, enabling cells to effectively utilize glucose for energy.
- A lack of sleep or poor sleep quality may lower insulin sensitivity, leading to insulin resistance and high blood sugar levels, all of which are risk factors for type 2 diabetes.

2. Glucose Metabolism:
- During sleep, the body performs critical metabolic activities such as glucose metabolism. Sleep deprivation or disruptions may disrupt these processes, resulting in poor glucose tolerance, elevated fasting blood glucose levels, and increased postprandial (after-meal) increases.
- Quality sleep promotes regulated hormone levels, including insulin, glucagon, cortisol, growth hormone, and leptin, which regulate blood sugar levels, hunger, energy balance, and metabolism.

3. **Hormonal regulation:**
- Sleep alters the release and balance of important hormones involved in glucose control. Adequate sleep, for example, aids in the regulation of cortisol levels, which may raise blood sugar levels when raised due to stress or sleep problems.
- Sleep deprivation may also influence ghrelin and leptin, hormones that govern hunger and fullness, resulting in increased appetite, desires for high-calorie meals, and disturbed eating habits, all of which can impair blood sugar management.

4. **Inflammation and Stress Responses:**
- Quality sleep helps to reduce inflammation and modulate the body's stress response. Chronic sleep deprivation or poor sleep quality may cause increased inflammation, oxidative stress, and sympathetic nervous system activation, all of which have a

deleterious influence on glucose management.
- Managing stress and fostering relaxation via enough sleep will help to minimize inflammation, stress-related blood sugar swings, and overall metabolic health.

5. **Energy balance and physical activity:**
- Good sleep improves energy balance, physical performance, and motivation for regular physical exercise. Adequate rest provides for appropriate recuperation, muscle regeneration, and energy restoration, allowing people to participate in physical activities that improve glucose metabolism.
- Sleep deprivation may cause weariness, lower exercise tolerance, decreased desire for physical activity, and disturbances in energy balance, all of which can impair insulin sensitivity and blood glucose management.

10 Tips for Improving Sleep Hygiene

Improving sleep hygiene entails developing healthy behaviors and establishing an atmosphere that promotes great sleep. Here are some useful recommendations for improving sleep hygiene and promoting peaceful, restorative sleep:

1. **Keep a Consistent Sleep Schedule.**
- Go to bed and get up at the same time every day, including weekends, to regulate your body's internal clock and develop a regular sleep-wake cycle.
- Consistency in sleep patterns optimizes circadian rhythms and promotes improved sleep quality over time.

2. **Plan a Relaxing Bedtime Routine:**
- Create a soothing pre-sleep ritual that tells your body it's time to unwind and prepare for sleep.

- Incorporate calming hobbies like reading a book, having a warm bath, deep breathing exercises, mild stretching, or listening to relaxing music.

3. **Optimize Your Sleep Environment**
- Keep your bedroom dark, quiet, and cold to promote good sleep. To block off light, use blackout curtains or eye masks, limit noise with earplugs or a white noise generator, and set the temperature to a comfortable level.
- Purchase a comfortable mattress, supporting pillows, and breathable bedding to improve sleep quality and encourage restful sleep.

4. **Limit Screen Time Before Bedtime:**
- Avoid using electronic devices like cell phones, tablets, laptops, and televisions at least an hour before bedtime, since the blue light generated by screens may

disrupt melatonin synthesis and interfere with sleep onset.
- Use a blue light filter on your electronic devices or night mode settings to minimize screen brightness in the evening.

5. **Monitor Your Diet and Hydration:**
- Avoid big meals, heavy snacks, caffeine, nicotine, and alcohol close to bedtime since they may impair digestion, increase alertness, and compromise sleep quality.
- Choose light, easily digested snacks as required, and remain hydrated during the day, but limit fluid consumption in the hours preceding up to sleep to decrease nightly awakenings.

6. **Perform Regular Physical Activity:**
- Incorporate regular physical activity into your daily routine, but try to finish strenuous exercise sessions earlier in the

day, since late-night exercise might stimulate and delay sleep onset.
- Moderate exercise, such as walking, yoga, or light stretching, may help you relax, decrease tension, and sleep better.

7. **Managing Stress and Anxiety:**
- Use stress-reduction strategies like mindfulness meditation, deep breathing exercises, progressive muscle relaxation, guided imagery, or journaling to quiet the mind, reduce anxiety, and promote relaxation before going to bed.
- Establish a worry-free nighttime routine by addressing problems early in the day and utilizing relaxation techniques to fall asleep comfortably.

8. **Limit napping throughout the day:**
- If you nap during the day, keep it brief (20-30 minutes) and avoid sleeping late in the afternoon or evening, since extended or late naps may interfere with

overnight sleep and disturb your sleep-wake cycle.

9. **Create a Comfortable Sleeping Environment:**
- Wear comfortable sleepwear, adjust the lighting to your liking (dim or soft), and utilize comfy bedding to create a nice and welcoming sleep environment that encourages relaxation and peaceful sleep.

10. **Seek Professional Help If Required:**
- If you continue to have persistent sleep problems, insomnia, sleep disorders, or difficulty falling or staying asleep despite good sleep hygiene, consult a healthcare professional, such as a sleep specialist or a sleep medicine provider.

By adopting these ideas into your daily routine and prioritizing sleep hygiene, you may increase sleep quality, relax more, optimize your sleep environment, and promote general well-being and health. Consistent practice of healthy sleep hygiene routines may result in improved sleep quality, energy levels, mood, and cognitive performance throughout the day.

Establishing a nighttime routine for improved sleep

A bedtime routine is a set of relaxing actions and behaviors you undertake before going to bed to communicate to your body that it's time to relax and prepare for restful sleep. Establishing a regular nighttime routine might help you sleep better, relax more, and feel better overall. Here are the stages of developing an effective nighttime routine for improved sleep:

1. **Establish A Consistent Bedtime:**
- Set a regular bedtime that allows for 7-9 hours of undisturbed sleep, taking

into account your sleep demands and routine.
- Try to go to bed and get up at the same time every day, including weekends, to regulate your body's internal clock and develop a regular sleep-wake cycle.

2. **Start winding down early:**
- Start your evening ritual at least 30 minutes to an hour before your target sleep time to allow for a smooth transition from awake to sleepy.
- Avoid stimulating activities or screen time close to bedtime, since these might disrupt melatonin synthesis and postpone sleep onset.

3. **Dim the Lights to Create a Relaxing Atmosphere.**
- Dim the lights in your bedroom or use soft, warm lighting to create a calming and relaxing atmosphere.
- Aromatherapy using essential oils like lavender, chamomile, or cedarwood may help you relax and feel peaceful.

4. **Take part in relaxing activities:**
- Select soothing activities that will help you unwind and relax, such as reading a book, listening to peaceful music, doing mild yoga or stretching, having a warm bath, or doing deep breathing exercises.
- Avoid exciting or intellectually taxing activities that may cause alertness and make it difficult to fall asleep.

5. **Practice mindfulness or meditation:**
- Incorporate mindfulness meditation or guided relaxation activities into your sleep routine to clear your mind, decrease tension, and promote inner peace.
- As you prepare to sleep, focus on deep breathing, body awareness, and letting go of rushing thoughts or anxieties.

6. **Limit Screen Time and Blue Light Exposure:**

- Avoid using electronic devices like cell phones, tablets, laptops, and televisions at least an hour before bedtime since the blue light generated by screens suppresses melatonin synthesis and disrupts sleep.
- Use night mode settings or blue light filters on your smartphone to lower screen brightness and blue light exposure in the evening.

By adding these actions into your nighttime routine regularly, you may create a peaceful and favorable atmosphere for better sleep, improve sleep quality, increase relaxation, and boost overall health. Adjust your bedtime routine depending on what works best for you, and try out various activities to discover a mix that helps you relax and prepare for a restful sleep every night.

CHAPTER 8

MONITORING & TRACKING

Monitoring and monitoring are critical components of efficient blood sugar control because they give useful insights into your glucose levels, help discover trends, and influence decisions about nutrition, exercise, medication, and lifestyle changes. Here's a detailed guide to efficiently monitoring and tracking blood sugar levels:

1. **Blood glucose monitoring:**
- Use a glucometer or continuous glucose monitoring (CGM) device to test blood glucose levels at different times of day, such as fasting (before meals), postprandial (after meals), bedtime, and as directed by a healthcare provider.
- Keep a journal, smartphone app, or digital spreadsheet of blood glucose readings to document trends, patterns, and changes over time.

2. **Tracking Meal Impact:**
- Maintain a food journal or use nutrition monitoring software to document your meals, snacks, portion sizes, carbohydrate intake, protein content, fat consumption, and meal scheduling.
- Take note of how various foods and meals influence your blood sugar levels, particularly any post-meal spikes or changes, and alter your eating patterns appropriately.

3. **Physical activity tracking:**
- Use a fitness tracker, pedometer, smartphone app, or wearable gadget to monitor your physical activity, workout routines, duration, intensity, and frequency.
- Keep track of how exercise affects your blood sugar levels, insulin sensitivity, and general health, and make adjustments to your activity schedule as appropriate.

4. **Medical Adherence:**
- Keep note of medication dosages, dosing schedules, insulin injections (if necessary), adherence to treatment programs, and any drug or dosage adjustments.
- Follow your healthcare provider's instructions, set medication reminders or alarms, and discuss any concerns or side effects with your healthcare team.

5. **Symptom monitoring:**
- Be aware of physical symptoms or indicators of blood sugar imbalances, such as frequent urination, increased thirst, lethargy, blurred vision, dizziness, mood swings, or hypoglycemia or hyperglycemia.
- Report any odd symptoms or changes in health status to a healthcare expert for examination and treatment.

6. **Emotional Wellbeing Tracking:**

- Keep track of your emotional well-being, stress levels, mood swings, sleep quality, energy levels, and general psychological wellness.
- Use stress-reduction tactics, relax regularly, prioritize decent sleep, and seek help from mental health specialists or support groups when necessary.

7. **Regular Check-Ups and Laboratory Tests:**
- Schedule frequent check-ups, follow-up consultations, and lab testing (e.g., HbA1c, lipid profile, kidney function tests) as directed by your healthcare practitioner.
- Examine lab results, consult with healthcare providers, and update treatment regimens or lifestyle modifications based on the most recent data.

8. **Pattern Recognition and Analysis:**

- Examine your monitoring data, such as blood glucose levels, meal impact, physical activity levels, medication adherence, symptoms, and emotional well-being, for patterns, trends, and connections.
- Look for trends linked to meal timing, carbohydrate consumption, exercise effects, medication efficacy, stresses, sleep problems, and other variables impacting blood sugar management.

9. **Goal-setting and Progress Tracking:**
- Establish clear, quantifiable goals for blood sugar control, HbA1c levels, weight management, exercise, dietary modifications, stress reduction, and other wellness objectives.
- Monitor progress toward your objectives, analyze accomplishments, celebrate milestones, and make changes to your action plans or tactics as appropriate.

10. **Collaborate with the Healthcare Team.**
- Present monitoring data, logs, and progress reports to your healthcare team during visits or consultations.
- Work with physicians, nurses, dietitians, diabetes educators, pharmacists, and other healthcare experts to get tailored advice, treatment modifications, education, and support.

By regularly monitoring and analyzing essential components of blood sugar control, you may obtain useful insights, make educated choices, discover areas for improvement, and enhance your overall glucose health. Stay proactive, and organized, and utilize technology, tools, and resources to help you monitor successfully. Regular monitoring enables you to take charge of your health, avoid issues, and meet your wellness objectives.

- The significance of frequent blood sugar monitoring (for diabetes patients)

The significance of regular blood sugar monitoring for diabetic individuals.

Regular blood sugar monitoring is critical in diabetes care because it helps you stay healthy, avoid problems, and achieve glucose control. Here are the main reasons why diabetics need to test their blood sugar regularly:

1. **Optimizing Glucose Management:**
- Regular monitoring enables diabetics to follow their blood sugar levels throughout the day and make educated food, medication, exercise, and lifestyle choices.
- By maintaining blood sugar levels within goal ranges, people may improve glucose control, lower their risk of hyperglycemia (high blood sugar) and hypoglycemia (low blood sugar), and enhance their general well-being.

2. **Preventing complications:**
- Keeping blood sugar levels within specified limits lowers the risk of long-term consequences from diabetes, such as cardiovascular disease, neuropathy, retinopathy, renal disease, and foot difficulties.
- Early identification of blood sugar swings or irregularities enables prompt interventions, medication changes, and preventative steps to reduce the severity of diabetes-related problems.

3. **Adjusting treatment plans:**
- Blood sugar monitoring gives essential data to healthcare practitioners, allowing them to evaluate treatment efficacy, change medication doses, and tailor diabetes management strategies.
- Monitoring findings enable healthcare practitioners to adjust treatment plans, insulin regimens, oral drugs, nutritional advice, and lifestyle interventions to

individual requirements and responses to therapy.

4. Understanding Patterns and Trends:
- Regular monitoring enables people to discover patterns, trends, and variables that influence blood sugar levels, such as meal timing, exercise effects, stresses, medication adherence, and time of day.
- By spotting trends, people may make specific modifications to their diet, exercise regimen, medication schedule, stress management strategies, and sleep habits to enhance glucose control and stability.

5. **Promoting self-management and empowerment:**
- Blood sugar monitoring enables diabetics to actively control their health, increase self-awareness, and make educated decisions about their daily activities and lifestyle choices.
- Monitoring blood sugar levels promotes accountability, incentive, and

responsibility for sticking to treatment regimens, implementing healthy habits, and reaching wellness objectives.

6. **Detecting hypoglycemia or hyperglycemia:**
- Regular monitoring detects hypoglycemia (low blood sugar) or hyperglycemia (high blood sugar) early, allowing for appropriate treatments, corrective measures, and symptom management.
- Recognizing and treating blood sugar imbalances as soon as possible helps to avoid problems, lowers the risk of severe hypoglycemia crises, and ensures safety and well-being.

7. ** Facilitating Communication with the Healthcare Team:**
- Monitoring data gives useful information for talks with healthcare practitioners during appointments, consultations, or telemedicine sessions.

- Sharing monitoring data, trends, difficulties, and accomplishments enables collaborative decision-making, tailored suggestions, and continuing support from the healthcare team.

In conclusion, regular blood sugar monitoring is critical for diabetics to improve glucose control, prevent complications, adjust treatment plans, understand patterns, promote self-management, detect blood sugar imbalances, facilitate communication with healthcare providers, track progress, and celebrate accomplishments. Individuals who prioritize frequent monitoring as part of diabetic self-care may improve their quality of life, lower the risk of complications, and attain long-term well-being.

- Keeping a diet and mood journal to monitor improvement.

Using a Food and Mood Diary to Monitor Progress

Keeping a food and mood journal is an effective tool for monitoring progress, discovering trends, and learning about how nutrition, emotions, and general well-being affect blood sugar levels and glucose control. Here's how to keep a food and mood journal effectively:

1. **Select A Format:**
- Choose the appropriate diary format for you, such as a physical journal, a digital app, a spreadsheet, or a notepad. Choose a format that is handy, accessible, and straightforward to utilize regularly.

2. **Record Your Food Intake:**
- Record or record all foods and drinks taken throughout the day, including meals, snacks, portion sizes, ingredients, cooking techniques, and any additional sauces or toppings.

- Include information such as carbohydrate composition, protein sources, fat sources, fiber-rich meals, and sugar content to better understand how various nutrients affect blood sugar levels.

3. **Note the Meal Timing:**
- Keep track of when meals and snacks are eaten, as well as the intervals between them. Pay attention to how meal time affects blood sugar levels, insulin sensitivity, and hunger signals.

4. **Tracking Blood Sugar Levels:**
- Record blood sugar measurements before and after meals, fasting blood glucose levels, postprandial (after-meal) rises, nighttime readings, and any other readings indicated by healthcare specialists.
- Take note of any symptoms or indicators of blood sugar swings, such as weariness, thirst, hunger, changes in mood, or physical pain.

5. **Monitor Emotional Wellbeing:**
- Make a column in your journal to record your feelings, moods, stress levels, energy levels, sleep quality, and general mental health throughout the day.
- Keep track of what influences your mood, such as stresses, activities, social interactions, exercise, sleep length, and coping methods.

6. **Describe the Eating Environment.**
- Describe the eating environment, context, and circumstances around meals and snacks, including where you ate, who you were with, how you felt, and any distractions or emotions you experienced.
- Be aware of emotional eating triggers, mindless eating habits, and eating patterns in reaction to stress, boredom, loneliness, or other emotional states.

7. **Review Patterns and Trends:**

- Review your food and mood diaries regularly to look for patterns, trends, correlations, and links between food choices, emotional states, blood sugar levels, and general well-being.
Look for trends in meal impact, carbohydrate consumption, emotional eating, stress reactions, blood sugar swings, energy levels, sleep quality, and mood changes.

Keeping a food and mood journal allows you to acquire useful insights, measure progress, make educated choices, discover areas for development, and enhance your blood sugar control and general well-being. Consistent monitoring and reflection enable you to take charge of your health, make good changes, and meet your glycemic and mental wellness objectives.

- Using technology (apps, wearable devices) to monitor health metrics

Using Technology (Apps, Wearable Devices) to Track Health Metrics

Technology has transformed health monitoring by giving simple tools, applications, and wearable devices that allow people to monitor a variety of health indicators such as blood sugar levels, physical activity, diet, sleep patterns, stress levels, and general well-being. Here's how to use technology successfully to measure health metrics:

1. **Select Relevant Apps and Devices.**
- Discover a variety of health and wellness applications for smartphones, tablets, and desktops that include tools for blood sugar monitoring, diet planning, exercise routines, sleep quality, stress management, and mood tracking.
Consider wearable gadgets like fitness trackers, smartwatches, blood glucose meters, continuous glucose monitoring (CGM) systems, and other connected

devices that work with health applications to gather data seamlessly.

2. **Tracking Blood Sugar Levels:**
- Use blood glucose monitoring apps or devices to check blood sugar levels throughout the day, such as fasting levels, pre-meal levels, postprandial levels (after meals), sleep readings, and any other readings indicated by healthcare providers.
- Connect blood glucose meters or CGM systems to compatible applications to automatically record data, see trends, produce reports, and share them with healthcare practitioners for analysis and advice.

3. **Track Nutrition and Meal Planning:**
- Use nutrition monitoring applications to register food intake, measure macronutrients (carbohydrates, proteins, and fats), monitor calorie consumption, record meal timing, and

analyze the effect of meals on blood sugar levels.
- Look into meal planning applications that include tailored meal ideas, recipes, portion management assistance, carbohydrate counting tools, and meal scheduling suggestions to help you manage your glucose levels.

4. **Log Physical Activity and Exercise:**
- Wear fitness trackers or smartwatches to measure your physical activity, including steps, distance traveled, calories burnt, heart rate, and exercise duration.
- Use exercise monitoring applications to record workouts, monitor exercise performance, establish fitness goals, get real-time feedback, and access guided workouts or training programs based on your fitness level and preferences.

Setting realistic blood sugar management targets.

Setting realistic goals for blood sugar control.

Setting realistic objectives is critical for maintaining good blood sugar management and overall glucose health. Setting attainable goals allows you to measure progress, remain inspired, and create long-term improvements to your well-being. Here's how to create realistic blood sugar management goals:

1. **Assess your current status:**
- Start by evaluating your current blood sugar levels, living habits, eating patterns, physical activity, stress, and general health.
- Use blood sugar monitoring instruments, such as glucose meters, to measure your blood glucose levels throughout the day and spot patterns or trends.

2. **Understanding Your Target Range:**

- Speak with healthcare experts, such as physicians, dietitians, or diabetes educators, to determine your target blood sugar range based on your age, health condition, medical history, and particular glucose control objectives.
- Learn about target blood sugar levels for fasting, pre-meal, post-meal, and nighttime readings to help you create goals.

3. **Identify Areas of Improvement:**
- Determine whether aspects of your lifestyle or behaviors may influence blood sugar control, such as nutrition, physical exercise, stress management, medication adherence, sleep quality, and hydration.
- Take into account carbohydrate intake, meal timing, portion sizes, sugar consumption, alcohol use, medication doses, and stress levels, all of which may need change.

4. **Set specific, measurable goals:**

- Establish clear, quantifiable blood sugar management targets, such as meeting target blood glucose levels before meals, lowering post-meal increases, improving fasting blood sugar levels, or maintaining consistent readings throughout the day.
- Track progress and assess achievement using quantitative metrics such as blood glucose readings (e.g., in mg/dL or mmol/L), HbA1c levels, or daily glucose fluctuation.

5. **Divide goals into manageable steps:**
- Divide major objectives into smaller, more achievable tasks or milestones that may be completed gradually over time. This method reduces overload and allows for gradual development.
- For example, if you want to limit post-meal blood sugar increases, start with one meal per day or make particular dietary modifications to lower glycemic index items.

6. **Set realistic timeframes:**
- Set realistic timescales for attaining your objectives based on your existing health, willingness to change, lifestyle restrictions, and capacity to adopt new behaviors.
- Avoid establishing too ambitious or unreasonable deadlines, which may lead to irritation and disappointment. Instead, promote incremental, long-term reforms.

Individuals who use digital tools, applications, and wearable devices to measure health data may obtain useful insights, remain motivated, establish attainable goals, monitor progress, and make educated choices to enhance their overall health, well-being, and quality of life. Consistent use of technology for health monitoring increases self-awareness, fosters responsibility, and enables people to make proactive efforts toward optimum well-being.

CHAPTER 9

LIFESTYLE CHANGES FOR LONG-TERM SUCCESS IN GLUCOSE MANAGEMENT

Long-term success in glucose health necessitates making permanent lifestyle adjustments that encourage balanced blood sugar levels, minimize cravings, and improve general well-being. Here are the important lifestyle modifications to concentrate on for long-term success:

1. **Healthy Food Habits:**
- Eat more entire, unprocessed foods, such as fruits, vegetables, whole grains, lean meats, and healthy fats.
- Limit your consumption of added sugars, sugary drinks, refined carbs, and processed meals, which may cause blood sugar spikes and cravings.

- Use portion management, thoughtful eating, and balanced meals to keep blood sugar constant throughout the day.

2. **Regular physical activity:**
- Include regular exercise in your regimen, aiming for a mix of aerobic, strength, flexibility, and balance activities.
- Select activities that you love and can continue over time to increase insulin sensitivity, boost glucose absorption by muscles, and support overall metabolic health.

3. **Stress management:**
- Prioritize stress-reduction activities including meditation, deep breathing, yoga, mindfulness practices, and relaxation exercises to reduce stress-related blood sugar swings and emotional eating.
- Maintain a good work-life balance by setting realistic objectives, delegating

chores, and practicing self-care to minimize stress and increase overall well-being.

4. **Quality Sleep:**
- Get enough sleep every night, aiming for 7-9 hours of quality sleep to support hormone control, metabolic function, and glucose metabolism.
- Create a regular sleep schedule, a calming nighttime habit, and an optimal sleep environment to promote restful sleep.

5. **Hydration:**
- Stay hydrated all day by drinking lots of water. Proper hydration improves kidney function, assists digestion, and regulates blood sugar levels.
- Avoid sugary beverages and instead drink water, herbal teas, or infused water with natural tastes to stay hydrated.

6. **Mindful Technology Usage:**

- Use technology wisely by limiting screen time, particularly before bedtime, to enhance sleep quality and decrease stress.
- Use health and wellness applications, wearable gadgets, and internet tools to monitor progress, remain inspired, and receive useful glucose-related information.

7. **Regular Monitoring and Checkups:**
- Monitor blood sugar levels regularly, as recommended by healthcare specialists. Keep track of trends, alter your lifestyle as required, and share any concerns or changes with your healthcare provider.
- Set up frequent check-ups, screenings, and meetings with healthcare practitioners, dietitians, and experts to evaluate general health, track progress, and get individualized advice.

8. **Social support and accountability:**
- Surround yourself with helpful friends, family, or support groups that promote healthy behaviors, motivate you, and hold you accountable.
- Communicate your objectives, problems, and accomplishments to others, seek advice and direction as required, and enjoy triumphs together.

9. **Educational Resources and Continuous Learning:**
- Stay informed and educated about glucose health, nutrition, exercise, stress management, and general wellness by reading trustworthy books, and articles, attending seminars, and taking online courses.
- Maintain your curiosity, openness to new knowledge, and willingness to change your lifestyle in response to evidence-based suggestions and personal experiences.

10. Consistency and Persistence:
- Adopt a long-term perspective and commit to continuous, sustainable lifestyle adjustments to achieve long-term glycemic health success.
- Be patient, persistent, and resilient while facing obstacles, setbacks, and temptations. Instead of striving for perfection, focus on making progress and celebrating minor triumphs.

By incorporating these lifestyle changes into your daily routine and thinking, you may lay the groundwork for long-term success in glucose management, greater well-being, and a healthier, more vibrant life. Remember that every good decision you make improves your overall health and quality of life, and your commitment to wellness is an investment in your future.

CONCLUSION

In conclusion, controlling blood sugar levels and minimizing cravings are critical components of achieving maximum health and wellness. Throughout this tutorial, we've looked at crucial tactics for improving glucose control and managing cravings successfully. Let's review a few of these major strategies:

1. **Balanced Diet:** Aim for a balanced diet high in complex carbs, lean proteins, healthy fats, fiber, and nutrient-dense foods. To avoid blood sugar spikes and cravings, limit your sugar consumption and avoid processed carbs.

2. **Regular Physical Activity:** Incorporate regular exercise into your regimen to enhance insulin sensitivity, boost glucose absorption by muscles,

and help with overall blood sugar management.

3. **Stress Management:** Use stress-reduction strategies including meditation, deep breathing, yoga, and relaxation exercises to reduce stress-induced blood sugar swings and emotional eating.

4. **Healthy Lifestyle Habits:** To keep blood sugar levels constant and avoid cravings, prioritize proper sleep, hydration, portion management, mindful eating, and consistent meal scheduling.

5. **Mindful Eating:** Pay attention to hunger signals, taste flavors, chew gently, and minimize distractions throughout meals to improve satisfaction and reduce overeating.

6. **Blood Sugar Monitoring:** To attain optimum glucose health, monitor

blood sugar levels regularly, follow physician advice, and make changes to your diet and lifestyle.

Encouragement to Maintain Commitment to Glucose Health: Maintaining glycemic health needs consistent effort, focus, and deliberate decisions. By following the tactics provided in this book and maintaining healthy behaviors, you may see long-term gains in blood sugar management, energy levels, and general well-being. Remember that little, beneficial adjustments build up over time, and every step toward glucose wellness represents a healthier, more vibrant existence.

Celebrate your accomplishments, keep inspired, and seek help from healthcare experts, nutritionists, and wellness groups as necessary. Your dedication to glycemic health is an investment in your long-term vitality and quality of life.

Continue to prioritize your health, listen to your body, and practice a balanced approach to diet and well-being. With effort and determination, you may reach your objectives of maintaining regulated blood sugar levels, reducing cravings, and promoting glucose health.

Here's to your ongoing success and well-being as you work toward glycemic wellness!